# Chance and Little Star

# Praise for Storyshares

"One of the brightest innovators and game-changers in the education industry."
– Forbes

"Your success in applying research-validated practices to promote literacy serves as a valuable model for other organizations seeking to create evidence-based literacy programs."
- Library of Congress

"We need powerful social and educational innovation, and Storyshares is breaking new ground. The organization addresses critical problems facing our students and teachers. I am excited about the strategies it brings to the collective work of making sure every student has an equal chance in life."
– Teach For America

"It's the perfect idea. There's really nothing like this. I mean, wow, this will be a wonderful experience for young people."
- Andrea Davis Pinkney, Executive Director, Scholastic

"Reading for meaning opens opportunities for a lifetime of learning. Providing emerging readers with engaging texts that are designed to offer both challenges and support for each individual will improve their lives for years to come. Storyshares is a wonderful start."
- David Rose, Co-founder of CAST & UDL

# Chance and Little Star

### Joseph Legaspi

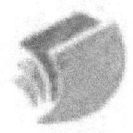

A Storyshares book

Storyshares

Story Share, Inc.

24 N. Bryn Mawr Avenue #340

Bryn Mawr, PA 19010-3304

www.storyshares.org

*Inspiring reading with a new kind of book.*

**Interest Level:** High School

**Grade Level Equivalent:** 2.5

9798885979221

Book design by Storyshares

Storyshares Presents

# Chapter One
# Blackout

*I COULDN'T BREATHE.*

I didn't understand what was going on. I only knew something was wrong.

I was sixteen then. I could've been sixty and still not known what was happening to me.

That was all I remembered before I fell asleep. Well, I thought I was asleep. I don't even remember that part. I think I was asleep because it felt like being asleep.

The doctors called it a "coma." Just that word scared me.

But there was something even more scary. They didn't know why I couldn't breathe. It could happen again.

And it did.

It was a month later. One minute, I was in my bedroom getting dressed for school. My mom was calling me from the kitchen.

"Kristena, is your school bag ready?"

The next minute, I was back in the hospital. Instead of my mom's voice, a stranger was saying, "Kristena, just breathe slowly."

The doctors ran more tests. It was useless. They still didn't know why I couldn't breathe.

Do you think it happened again?

It sure did.

With each new episode I grew more sad and more scared.

It bothered my parents as much as it bothered me. It also made them act weird. They started asking a lot more questions after they brought me home from the hospital. They kept asking how I was feeling.

My teachers and pals at school asked me that same thing.

A few kids asked what exactly was wrong with me.

I didn't mind what other people said. At least, that's what I told myself at the start. I thought it was nice of them to ask. But it made me embarrassed too, not being able to explain myself.

Each time I went to the hospital, my mom held my hand the whole night. My dad was there too. He would give me *his* hand when my mom was tired.

On my third visit, Dad was talking to someone at the hospital about some papers. I overheard them mentioning money. Dad's face didn't look happy.

I looked at my mom, sitting at the side of my bed. I asked her, "Does dad have enough to pay the doctors?"

Mom rubbed my chest and simply said, "Don't worry. Just relax. It'll be ok."

It wasn't. They didn't have enough and needed to save money.

A few weeks later, we moved from the Upper West Side into a neighborhood called Helwick. It's the part of New York City where apartment rooms are smaller and older. They are dirtier and more crowded too. Graffiti is everywhere.

My parents tried to hide it from me. But I wasn't stupid. We had moved to the poorer part of the city. The air smelled bad. People didn't look happy there.

Helwick wasn't where I wanted to live. And the worst part was that it was all my fault.

Late one night, my parents heard me crying and rushed to my room.

"It's my fault. I'm sorry," I cried. I pulled out my hair until my scalp started to bleed.

"No," my parents said. "Don't blame yourself. We're going to get you the right help. We won't stop until you get better. We promise."

Over the next several weeks, I went to more doctor offices than I want to remember. They were all the same, except one. I didn't notice the difference at first. But that's how life went for me. It was full of surprises.

# Chapter Two

# The Painting

IT WAS A WEDNESDAY morning. My homeroom teacher passed me a note from someone named William H. Toussaint. He had these letters after his name: PhD and PsyD.

The note told me to meet Dr. Toussaint this afternoon. It was scribbled with a sloppy drawing of the school building that showed how to get to his office. It was on the top floor by the corner, far from the usual busyness of the school.

When I came to Dr. Toussaint's door, it was wide open, but the small office was dark. The blinds were shut. The only light came from a tiny desk lamp. It gave the room a warm glow.

A man with a short beard was sitting behind a desk, writing. He was wearing small, silver-framed glasses and a brown jacket. His tie seemed too small for him.

"Kristena?" the man behind the desk said. He looked up briefly at me, his pen still moving.

"Yes," I said, looking in slowly with my head. The rest of my body was still in the doorway.

"Don't be afraid. Come in," he said. "Have a seat. I'll be with you in a second."

Dr. Toussaint seemed to be signing papers. He was writing something short and swift on every page.

I looked around the office.

Small plants were hanging above us. On his window sill, there was a football-sized rock. On the wall behind his desk was a brightly colored painting. It was a giant butterfly. Next to that was another painting of a little girl dressed in a white Easter bonnet. She wore a sad expression on her face. Dr. Toussaint looked up for a moment and caught me staring at that painting.

"Do you like Monet?" he asked.

"Who?"

"Claude Monet was the artist for that painting. Really something, isn't it?" He put down his pen and took off his glasses. "So," he said,

"how are you?"

He reached out his hand as he moved to the other chair in front of the desk. He sat just a few inches away from me.

"I'm fine," I replied. I pushed my chair back a little.

He smiled. We were silent for a few seconds.

"Kris-teen-a. Am I pronouncing that right?" he asked politely.

"Kris-ten-a," I corrected him, emphasizing the short vowel sound in the middle.

"I'm sorry," he said. "You must get a lot of people who mispronounce your name."

"Yeah, but it's a weird name," I admitted. "Most people just call me Kristen. No 'a' at the end. The ones who remember my full name mispronounce it as Christina. At least they all get the 'Kris' part right."

Dr. Toussaint put on his glasses and read something in the folder on his lap. "I see you skipped two grades. Once in elementary school. Again in middle school. Now, you're one year away from starting college when most kids are just getting used to high school. Wow, this is really something!"

"I blame it on my math scores," I said.

He lifted his head when I said that. "Interesting that you put it like that," he said, with a tilt of his head. "It's great that you love math so much."

We were silent again.

"Can you tell me a little more about yourself, Kristena?" Dr. Toussaint eventualy asked.

I looked at my watch. "How much longer until I can get back to class?"

"Why the rush?"

"I have a math quiz," I said. "I just need to know what's wrong with me. Can you tell me?"

"First I need to know a bit more about you."

"Ok, well, what do you want to know?" I asked, looking at my watch again.

"Don't worry about that quiz. Tell me anything," he said. "What do you usually tell people when they first meet you?"

"Well, my mom is Irish Catholic. We don't eat meat on Fridays. It's weird because I love steak and so does my dad," I said. "He isn't religious. He's from Japan. They sorta meet in the tea. They both love tea, but I drink juice."

Dr. Toussaint laughed.

"My mom can't handle chopsticks, but my dad doesn't like forks and spoons," I said.

"Was it hard growing up with two cultures?" he asked.

"Why are you asking all these questions about my parents?" I asked him.

"I'm simply trying to get to know you better. Tell me more," he prompted.

"My mom is good at Irish dancing. She tried to teach my dad but he wasn't into it as much," I said.

He nodded.

"Look, I know why I'm here," I said. "I gotta ask again. Can you fix me?"

"We'll get to that," Dr. Toussaint promised. "For now, I just want us to get to know each other. Is that ok?"

I nodded and looked again at the painting of the little girl.

We talked about his love of art. He told me some stories about his other hobby, fishing.

He asked me what I like to do besides math. I told him I like reading.

All in all, I actually enjoyed that first chat with him. He was nice, but still, it didn't help. I was beginning to hope I was getting better, but... then I couldn't breathe again.

# Chapter Three
# The Reading

THE TRIP TO THE hospital was worse this time. They took me to the part of the hospital for the sickest patients. They ran more advanced tests. That was another word for more expensive tests.

*How could this happen again?* I felt like my world was starting to spin right on its axis again.

My dad was there to hold my hand through all the tests.

"Kristena, Kristena," my dad would whisper in my ear. "I love you very much." He repeated it over and over.

His tears were dripping on my cheek. It was like Niagara Falls. I felt like saying, "I love you too, Dad, but can you please use a tissue?"

The problem was that it was hard to speak. It was like my jaw muscles were locked. In fact, all my muscles were so tight I was like one big cramp.

My dad lost his job for being by my side so much. That didn't make my mom happy.

"I have to go to my new job now. Your mom will be here later when she gets off from work. See you tonight, my little star," my dad said.

My test results came back. They still couldn't find anything wrong. They were discharging me. I had to wait for my mom to come and take me home.

It was so boring just lying down in bed. I wandered around the halls until my mom came.

I saw many different patients. Some looked like they were in physical therapy. A few were on stretchers. Others were walking around like me. They were all kids. Some were older than me and some were younger. But they were all just kids.

In one large room, I overheard a young woman speaking in a lovely British accent. She was reading Emily Dickinson poems to a boy.

The boy had deep, dark brows and a strong, square jaw. His chin reminded me of the kind Superman or Batman has.

I kept listening to the woman read. It felt strange to hear such beautiful words. They didn't match this place. The only other sounds here were people coughing, groaning, and sometimes crying or screaming. The poetic sound of those words was so comforting.

She looked at me as I approached. When I sat down, I asked her,

"May I listen too?"

"Of course," she said. "We'd love a bigger audience. Right, Lam?" The boy didn't answer.

"I just love Emily Dickinson," I said. We started chatting about her poems. Then I asked the boy, "Do you like her poems too?"

"Oh, he doesn't speak," the woman said quietly. She explained that she was a volunteer who reads to patients.

The woman noticed the time and said she had to leave. She didn't realize it was so late.

"Any chance I can keep reading to him?" I asked.

"That would be great. His mom's around the corner. She'll be here soon." She turned to the boy and waved. "Bye, Lam!"

I saw another book on the table next to us. It was by Charles Dickens. I read that to Lam for a good ten minutes.

"I see you've met my dashing young gentleman," a woman interrupted. She was trying to imitate a British accent too. She wasn't as good with accents as the volunteer, but she had a friendly voice. She stroked the boy's hair. "How are you, Lam, my sweetheart?"

I noticed her kind eyes and light brown skin. They were just like her son's. She had straight, dark hair. Some of it was grey. Her long face was full of smiling wrinkles.

"I'm Kristena," I said.

"I'm Acia. Thanks so much for reading to him. He has a stack of books at home that I read to him every day." She looked at Lam and sighed.

Then her eyes looked up and down at my patient gown. "Oh my, how are you, dear? Are you ok?"

"Better. Thanks for asking," I said. "I'm being discharged soon."

"Awesome!" She gave me a big thumbs up. "Lam's little heart is giving us troubles again. But he's being discharged too. I just got his papers."

"That's awesome too! Well, nice to meet you both," I said.

Acia didn't seem like she wanted to leave.

"Kristena, you have such a lovely voice. Do you want to keep reading to Lam?" she asked.

"Yeah, I do," I answered.

I must have read for an hour. When I finally put the book down, Acia was still smiling.

"Thanks again, Kristena!" She put her hands together and clapped. "Lam and I sure loved your reading. I can tell from your voice that you love literature. You must read a lot!"

"Here and there... whenever I have the time," I said.

"There's a library near us that has readings of the classics every Tuesday. Lam and I are there each time. Front row! Come by, we'll save you a seat!" she said.

I actually did go to the library. After several visits, Acia even invited me to come to their home and read to Lam again myself.

# Chapter Four

# The Evening Home

ACIA AND LAM LIVED on the side of Brooklyn where big shadows fell. The biggest one came from a huge billboard. It was between their house and the Brooklyn Bridge.

Inside their house, the ceiling above was rosy-white. It was framed with silver lines. Dark red curtains with gold trim hung in all the windows. They were the thickest curtains I've ever seen. Tables were padded along the edges. Electrical sockets were filled with safety plugs, like there were small children in the house. Plants on the windows sat high and out of reach.

At the front door, I could already smell lemon broth and salty fish.

"Before you read, let's eat first!" Acia said, the instant she let me in.

Her eyes were so red. I thought it was probably from chopping onions. She took off a pink headband and quickly wiped her eyes with it. Then she opened up her long, skinny arms and hugged me so tightly. I could feel the heat and wetness of her apron.

Thick steam was rising from four large pots on the stove. A brown woven basket of apples sat in the center of the kitchen table.

Acia cooked so much food that I thought there were other people invited, like a party. But it was just the three of us. She dressed Lam in a handsome silk shirt. It was buttoned to the top and neatly tucked. I wondered if I was dressed too casually. I only had on a plain pink T-shirt and ripped jeans.

Acia's voice had great energy. She talked fast as she told me stories of growing up the Philippines.

She laughed hard too. In fact, she laughed so hard she had to wipe tears from her eyes.

After we ate, she led me to a room on the first floor. She gently opened the door and we walked in. Everything in the room was quiet, or turned quiet. The heavy carpet made our footsteps silent. It was a darker room than the living room and kitchen. Because it was so dark, it seemed bigger. Books were oddly tied together on shelves rising as high as the ceiling.

On a table near the bed was a smaller stack of books. Acia said those were Lam's favorite. The top one was his number one.

She sat Lam near the window in a rocking chair. It was padded and made of reddish-brown oak wood.

I read him several poems from Robert Frost and T.S. Eliot.

He soon fell asleep.

"Don't take it personally, Kristena," Acia said. She patted me on the shoulder. "Too much lemon broth. He had a good appetite tonight. That's what knocked him out."

A black blanket was folded neatly on Lam's lap. His eyes darted about as he slept. They were moving so fast. Lines under his eyes were rose-pink. They looked like the edges of clouds in a sunset.

Acia stared at him tenderly. She slowly shook her head, saying,

"Look at him, Kristena. If there ever was a child who loved to sleep..."

"Acia... Lam's never spoken in his life?" I asked.

I didn't think there was anything wrong with the question, but I quickly realized I shouldn't have asked it.

Acia covered her eyes. She bit her lower lip.

"I'm sorry, Acia. I didn't mean to—"

"Oh, please. It's not you." Acia put her hand on my arm. "Sometimes I get like this."

"I should go," I said.

"It's ok." Acia let out a tired sigh. "He grunts softly when he's hungry. He cries like a whimper when in pain. Other than that, he's got no language. None." Her voice pounded on each word. It exploded on the last.

She told me stories of taking Lam to speech therapists, doctors, and special schools. She even took him to monasteries in Tibet and healers in Africa and ashrams in India. Still, nobody could fix him.

Acia took one of the cotton sheets from his bed and draped it over Lam's tummy and legs.

"Lam was born crying so loud, you know," she whispered. "I thought I'd go deaf before I brought him home. Then, he slowly stopped. One day he became as silent as leaves falling. There's still a voice somewhere inside him. I know it. Whatever made him cry could also make him speak. Oh, Lam."

She swallowed and took another deep breath. "He's eighteen now. Oh, Kristena, I'd do anything to have him talk to me, even one word."

I didn't know what to say. Her face got even sadder in an instant. She rubbed my hand and all I thought to say was, "I'm so sorry."

"No, don't be sorry for us. Don't ever say that, Kristena. Never. Ok?" Acia said.

I thought I offended her even more. But her tone suddenly softened. She smiled and looked towards the kitchen. "More broth? More rice? Juice?"

"Thank you, but my mother might want me home now," I said. "If I may, I'd like to say goodnight to Lam before I go."

"Of course, dear," she said.

She led me back to his bedroom. We sat with him for a minute. We watched him sleep, staring at his tousled hair from his mother's repeated finger-combing. I thought of my mom touching my hair.

I almost caught his eyes blinking open, once or twice. I wondered if he was trying to say something. Questions came up in my mind. What was that thing holding him back from talking? Acia didn't know. It was the same as me not knowing what was choking me.

His pain must be the same as mine.

I understood completely.

I bid them goodnight.

It took me half an hour to get to my home. As I got close to my door, I could already see my mom in the dark hallway. The lights brightened when I came close. She pulled me in as soon as I opened the door.

"Why are you back so late? I was worried sick. Are you ok?" she asked.

I told her all about Acia and Lam. I had a lot to say. We ended up having hot cocoa and chatting for a long time. Then I remembered. I didn't finish my homework.

"It can wait," my mom said. "Catch up tomorrow. You need to go to bed now."

But I couldn't sleep that night. All I thought about was Lam. I tore off a sheet of loose-leaf paper and began to write.

*I am Lam. I am a boy. I am broken; I cannot speak or write to let you know how I feel. But here, in this place where feelings make things real, I can do that and much more. Sometimes I am aware of this place I am in. But often I am not. You happened to catch me in one of those moments when I know I am dreaming — dreaming in my sleep.*

*Does this also happen to you? I do not know, but I hope it happens to you a lot. To me, it feels so good. I feel like someone else here — someone happy.*

*Here, I can do anything! I want to be on the moon and I am there. I get tired of being there and I think about being back on earth. Then I am back here. Clouds and mountains and walls do not stop me. Sometimes nothing does. I can have almost everything I want.*

*Almost.*

*People in my dreams still do not hear me.*

*In every dream I am a little different. In one dream, I am six years old. In another, I am sixteen. Right now, I think I am about eighteen. But I do not know for sure.*

*Time. What is that? No one here knows what that is. I do not think they care. I do not care. I only know that I am here now.*

*Not all my dreams are as good as this one. Sometimes I can't control everything. And as much as I love this place, I would trade all the sleep in the world for the gift of telling you all this when I am awake.*

*Awake. Feeling awake. Being awake. Thinking awake. How does that feel? I want to know. It is too much for me, being awake in the world. Too many feelings break my heart. I am telling the truth. I cannot live in that real world.*

After writing, there was this peace that I can't describe. I fell asleep and it was a good, deep sleep.

# Chapter Five

## The Drive

AT MY NEXT SESSION with Dr. Toussaint, he was standing when I entered his office.

"Hello, Kristena, how are you today?" Dr. Toussaint asked. He rubbed his beard and sat down. "I haven't seen you for a while."

"Well... I was out," I said.

"Yes, you were in the hospital again." He paused. "You didn't want to tell me?"

I gave an unconcerned shrug, but straightened up in my seat.

"I didn't see the point," I said in a low voice.

"Point?" he asked.

"Yeah, I mean, you never mentioned my hospital visits last time we met," I said. "Isn't that why you're seeing me?"

"As I said, we'll get to that," he said.

I rolled my eyes.

"Well, how are things?" Dr. Toussaint asked.

"Ok," I answered.

"What have you been doing besides school work these past few weeks?" he asked.

"Writing," I replied.

"Really?" he asked. "Writing about what?"

"Just writing a lot lately. I did it a lot when I was little," I said.

"Why did you stop?" he asked.

"It's no big deal," I answered.

"Are you sure?" Dr. Toussaint asked.

"Yes," I said. "Can we talk about something else?"

"Ok, tell me whenever you're ready," he said. "What else do you want to talk about?"

"I don't know," I said.

"How about home life? Everything ok with mom and dad?" he asked.

"Yeah," I answered.

"Then how about school? The Assistant Principal says you haven't applied for some of the colleges on your list yet," he said. "He also told me that you're not handing in your homework lately, especially your math homework."

"Oh, ok, is this really why you wanted to see me? You want to talk about my grades?" I asked.

"Your grades are still above average," he said. "But I wonder if you could answer a very important question for me. What's driving you to study so hard?"

I was quiet, shifting my gaze to the window. "Why do you want to know?" I asked. I looked away at the door this time. I wondered: *if I ran out fast enough, what would Dr. Toussaint do?*

"Just curious," he said. He turned his eyes towards the door the same time I did. He moved his chair an inch closer to me and spoke

gently. "You know, everything we talk about here is strictly confidential. You don't have to be afraid. I won't tell anyone." "I'm not afraid, and I don't know what drives me," I lied to him.

"Ok?"

"Is there anything that is bothering you now?" he asked. "I don't mean just here in school."

"No. Not a thing. Everything is perfect. I'm perfect—or at least, trying to be," I said in an exasperated tone.

"Kristena, no one is perfect. In fact, most people who highly excel in one area are making up for a deficiency in another," Dr. Toussaint said.

"Deficient? What do I not have?" I asked.

"I was hoping you could tell me what that is," he said. "I'm very glad you are working so hard. All your teachers are. But sometimes work is a way we hide other things in our lives, painful things."

"I'm ok," I said.

"Good," he said. He stared at me and nodded.

"Really. I am," I said, putting on a smile. "I've never felt better."

Dr. Toussaint looked at me for a long time.

"Then why did you go to the hospital again?" he asked.

"I don't know. That's what I asked you before," I said. "Don't *you* know why?"

"I'll tell you what I really think," he said. "You seemed fine when we started to chat. But things changed when I brought up your writing and asked why you stopped when you were little. Now you sound defensive."

I didn't notice I was protecting something or trying to avoid the subject.

"Can I please go now?" I said. I was breathing heavily.

"Just relax, Kristena," Dr. Toussaint said.

"Please, I need to go! I'm missing a really important English class," I said.

"Don't worry about that. I spoke to your English teacher. You can pick up a copy of her notes in the office at the end of the day. I only have one more important question and then you're free to leave." Dr.

Toussaint folded his hands and said gently, "How do you feel about Mr. Narchese?"

"Mr. Narchese? My math teacher?" I wriggled in my seat again.

"What can I say?" I crossed my arms and stared at Dr. Toussaint.

"He got me the nomination for the College Math Scholars Program. Everyone's happy for me. Full scholarship!"

"Yes, congratulations," he said. "As I understand it, you'll need to choose Math as your major course of study in college. Do you feel pressured by it?"

"Not at all. Mr. Narchese said majoring in math can help me with a lot of stable careers, like accounting or scientific research. I'll make good money," I said.

"When you said that, your tone of voice sounded just like his. Please, tell me how *you* feel about that. *You*." Dr. Toussaint got more comfortable. He stretched his arms, made relaxing circular motions with his shoulders, and sat back patiently.

"I have nothing to say about it," I said in a quiet voice.

"Say anything," he said calmly. "Whatever pops into your head right now."

"Nothing," I said.

"You must be thinking of something," he said.

"Yeah, I'm thinking: why don't you just let me go to English class?" I asked.

"English class. I think I see now." Dr. Toussaint nodded, rubbing his beard. "Before I let you leave, I want you to remember I'm only here to help. I won't judge you. Ever. I will never tell anyone what you tell me about Mr. Narchese or anyone else. You understand this, correct?"

I nodded.

He looked down at the report on his lap. He opened it and briefly wrote something down.

"All right, you're free to leave," he said.

He wrote my name on the back of his business card. "I'm giving you my cell number. Call me if you ever feel stressed or need to talk about anything right away." He gave the card to me and said,

"Otherwise, I'll see you in two weeks."

# Chapter Six

# The Drawing

OVER THE NEXT FEW months, I visited Acia and Lam's house at least once a week after school. I went just to read to Lam. But of course, Acia always cooked up a feast.

Soon I was going there four times in two weeks. On the fourth night I asked Acia if she minded that I came so often.

"Nonsense," she said. "Good company is the best salt with any food."

Lam was always there. He was handsomely dressed by Acia in his best casual clothes. He was always in his rocking chair. He'd be staring into air. I couldn't prove it, but I thought he was staring at something there that no one else could see.

I was reading Lam my writing. Acia loved it.

In fact, Acia showed me something amazing.

She led me to Lam's room where his favorite books were stacked on the table. What was on top? It was my loose-leaf paper that I first wrote for him.

"I didn't put it there." Acia smiled widely. "He did!"

"Are you serious?" I asked.

"I kid you not." She glowed even brighter when she added, "Oooh, I think my little Lam has a big crush on you!"

I think it made me blush for the first time in my life.

She encouraged me to write some more and read it to Lam. So I wrote this story and read it to them at my next visit:

*A teacher was showing her class a stick figure of a man. It was drawn without any arms. She asked the class, "Children, do any of you see something wrong with this picture?"*

Everyone in the class said the picture wasn't finished, except one boy. "Nothing's wrong with the picture," he said.

The class laughed at him. The boy's mother had just suffered a stroke and was in a coma. They thought maybe he was stressed out and not thinking straight.

But the teacher looked curiously at the boy. She pointed him out and said, "Are you sure? Look closer."

The boy studied the picture and shrugged. "The man's face," he said.

"His face?" The teacher stared back at the picture.

"Yes," the boy said. "He has no eyes."

The teacher took a pen and put two dots on the figure for eyes. "Anything else wrong with this picture?" she asked.

The boy looked at the picture for a long time and said, "The man's shirt, I guess."

"His shirt?" the teacher asked. "What about his shirt?"

"No buttons," the boy said.

"All right," said the teacher. She drew two buttons on the figure. "Do you see anything else wrong?"

"Nope," the boy said.

"Nope?" The teacher finally gave up and said plainly to the boy, "What about his arms?"

"Well," said the boy, "he could have them behind his back."

The teacher challenged him even more and asked, "How do you know he had them behind his back? What if this person had no arms? Can you draw a person with no arms?" She held the picture up for the boy to look at again.

"Even if he had no arms," the boy said, "he's still a complete person."

Acia loved it. She remembered when Lam was bullied in preschool. She wished she could have read this story to the kids and teachers back then.

She said, "Other kids were making fun of him, trying to get him to talk. He should be treated like a regular person, just the same as everyone else. I told them whenever Lam did talk, the first thing he would probably say is, 'Shut up, you kids talk too much!'"

I smiled, and looked at Lam. "Yeah, that's what you should say, Lam."

# Chapter Seven

# The Teacher

"HELLO, KRISTENA, HOW ARE you today?" Dr. Toussaint asked. He was drinking a cup of coffee.

"Good," I said.

"You seem a bit more cheerful than usual," he observed, smiling at me.

"I met this quiet boy at the hospital. I've been having a lot of fun visiting his house," I said. "I read to him. He and his mother like it."

"Good for you. I'm glad you found something to do that's meaningful and fun," he said.

"I wrote this short story about bullying that they liked," I said.

"Interesting," he said. "Actually, I wanted to talk to you about that today."

"Is that why you mentioned Mr. Narchese last time?" I asked.

"I know his teaching method is a bit too rough for some kids," he said.

"I thought you said you don't reveal what others tell you," I said.

"I heard and saw it myself," Dr. Toussaint said. "He shouts when he teaches. We can all hear it. He thinks yelling and belittling students pushes them to work harder. I happen to disagree. Some may say it's bullying. But you seem to handle him very well. Have you ever dealt with anyone like him before?"

"A teacher?" I asked.

"Anyone," he said.

"Well... there was this teacher in kindergarten who hurt... no, I mean, he was tough with me," I admitted.

"You said 'hurt,'" Dr. Toussaint said.

"Did I?" I asked.

"Did he hurt you?" he asked. He looked me straight in the eyes.

"It was just a slip," I explained. "I didn't mean to say that."

"A slip of the tongue is often not a slip at all," he said with a tone of concern. "Let's talk more about him. How was he tough with you?"

"It was just something he said. No big deal," I said.

"But it hurt you," he said.

"Yeah, but the other kids said it was nothing," I said. "They said I was taking it too hard. Someday it'll go away."

I began to fidget and look at the door.

"I can see you did take it hard," Dr. Toussaint said. "It didn't go away, did it? It stayed with you until now. I can hear it in your voice." "It's just words," I said.

"Words can hurt just as deeply as anything else. Sometimes they leave scars inside us that last longer than cuts and bruises," he said.

I looked up at the painting of the little girl again.

"Can we talk about something else?" I asked.

"As always, I don't want to push you if you're not ready to talk about something. This sounds serious," he said. "Take your time.

But don't push this away. I want us to talk about this more. Again, I want you to feel safe here."

"I do," I said. I quickly grabbed my school bag. "See you next time."

I rushed out of his office faster than I ever did before.

# Chapter Eight

# Birthday

GOING TO ACIA'S HOUSE and warm kitchen table gave me the same excitement as a holiday, especially on Lam's birthday.

All year, Acia saved up every penny for the decorations and food. She stayed up the entire night to cook pots of pancit, which was long noodles mixed with shrimp, carrots, and sprouts. Acia told me that pancit was a Filipino tradition on birthdays for wishing long life.

I almost didn't recognize the living room. White streamers hung on the wall and blue balloons covered the ceiling. The design reminded me of a winter scene, with snow-covered branches against a bright, cloudless sky.

On the coffee table were flower and bird shapes carved out of melons. Acia also put up blinking colored lights all around the house, so in the evening it would look like Christmas.

In the kitchen, a shiny, white cake box sat in the center of the table. It was big enough to fit a TV inside, but the box was double the size of the small cake that hid in it.

On every table in the house, Acia put plenty of tall soda bottles, salty chips, and hot pancit. There was enough to feed a park full of children twice over.

Acia was pleasant in the morning, but she became uptight once the party started. She was hustling to socialize with guests and serve food. As more parents and children arrived, they kept their distance from Lam.

Left alone, Lam would often wander into the kitchen and spill soda or knock down a bowl. Sometimes Acia would throw a bowl too. She would scream, "Go ahead, Lam. Do it again. See me get really mad."

As I led Lam away, I could hear Acia give a long, tired sigh. It was almost a groan. She muttered to herself, "I'm not going to cry this year. I won't."

I told Acia I would watch Lam and she gave me a great big hug.

It was time to put the cake in front of Lam. With the lights out, everyone sang happy birthday. Acia blew out the candles.

Some children winced when they accidentally tapped Lam on the shoulder. Others moved away if they touched his hands. They had seen Lam act up before from the wrong touch, even if it was as light as the brush of cat's whiskers.

As hard as Acia tried to make this feel like a normal birthday party, it wasn't.

No one took pictures. The flash would be too much for Lam unless someone put on his sunglasses. But Acia wouldn't allow it on his birthday.

No hugs or kisses for Lam. No one clapped. No jokes or laughter. We even stood a little distance from him, our smiles unnoticed in the silent dark.

I heard some children pout and say to their mothers, "Can we go home now?" I turned to Acia as the lights came on. I smiled to cheer her, in case she heard it. But her red, tired, disappointed eyes looked teary.

She would cry again cleaning up, again putting Lam to bed, and again in the morning. This day was supposed to be special, but it would be another ordinary day for her.

When all the guests left, she said to me, "Thank you for smiling all day today."

"No worries," I said. "Why wouldn't I be happy for Lam?"

She explained, "On the day to celebrate life, the cruelest act is to be unhappy. If you're going to cry or take pity, do it alone. Don't come, even if it means no celebration. I've said that to guests in the past. Thankfully, not this year."

Before I left, I went to Lam's room. He was fast asleep.

"Happy Bornday, Lam. You're my coolest friend," I said. "Here's a birth-day poem I wrote for you. I don't know about tomorrow. I may breathe again, or not. If today is all I have, I'm glad I spent it with you. I hope you feel the same way on your special day. The poem is called 'Years.' See you next time."

*I had known you for more*

*Than three thousand*

*Rising and setting suns But it seemed like just one long waking moment* between sleep.

*And if it was only a day*

*I was yours for a day*

*As I know your wish is mine:*

*That the day never Touches the night.*

# Chapter Nine

# The Dance

IN THE LIVING ROOM Acia turned on an old stereo. Strauss' "The Blue Danube" started playing. Lam's hands began dancing. They were waltzing with the air, taking wild turns like a clumsy ballet performer. I saw a cute crinkle appear on the bridge of his pointy nose.

"My, oh my, Lam, what a wonderful mood you're in right now,"

Acia said. She stroked his hair and turned towards me. "You know, Kristena, he rarely smiles and he's smiling at you! How delightful!"

I looked at his eyes, then at his smile, then at his nose. The crinkle was deep.

Acia left the room and told me to watch Lam. She returned and handed me a bowl of vanilla ice cream, dressed with a little river of chocolate syrup and a baby banana on the side. I thanked her.

I kept watching Lam dance by himself until he plopped down on the floor. Acia brought two wicker baskets out of the closet. They were full of cowbells, bongos, hand-sized tambourines, maracas, wrist and hand bells. She carried them so fast I thought she'd throw them up in the air. We soon filled the living room with noisemaker sounds, like midnight on New Year's.

"Let it all out!" Acia cried. She was shaking a tambourine in one hand and maracas in the other. "No one can hear us here for miles."

We sat on the floor and filled the air with our sounds. I don't know how long we did that. It felt like a few hours. Acia ran to the basement every so often to get more noisemakers.

The last few days though, Lam didn't have as much energy as usual. Acia told me that all this time awake wasn't what he was used to. He'd only listen for a minute or two and stop. Sometimes he didn't even last for a minute.

So instead of dancing, Acia and Lam would just listen to me read.

Of course, we had our usual big dinners.

At one point, Acia talked about the past. "When I was little, I wanted to be a dancer," she said. "I stopped trying many times. I listened to others tell me I was no good. Why did I ever listen to them? Where are they now? Certainly not here. So what was the point of listening to them? The only one standing here is me. I am left here listening to my regrets. I let those people destroy my life."

"You know, Acia, I haven't applied to colleges yet. I was thinking of applying to a local writing school," I said. "One of their new teachers is a writer from Japan that I adore. But my math teacher will hate that. He manages a big college math scholarship program. He chose me out of hundreds of students. He'll be really disappointed."

"Just go for it. Remember us when you're famous!" She raised a glass to toast my future. "What masterpiece are you working on next for us?"

"I want to try a comedy piece. I don't know. What do you think?" I asked.

"Sure! We all need a laugh. We can't wait to hear it!" she said.

I had written something, but not finished it. I told Acia I was coming next week, but I decided to stop by the next day. I wanted to see what they thought of the first few lines.

When I arrived at their house the door was open, but oddly Acia wasn't there to greet me.

She was curled up on the living room floor. Her head was in her hands. Later I found out where she had been. She had just come back from the hospital.

Without looking up, she said softly, "Lam's heart again."

She shook her head and looked at me. She only said one word, but I could already tell from her face: "Gone."

I shook my head in disbelief. "No, no, no."

I came all cheerful and ready to make them laugh.

I had no idea this would be the saddest day of my young life.

# Chapter Ten

# Recovery

Dr. Toussaint got up and took a tissue from a box on his desk. He gave it to me and moved his chair closer.

"I'm very sorry," he said. "I know I can never feel the amount of pain you do, but I can understand your suffering."

"No you don't. You can't. Stop pretending you're me. You're not me, ok?" I said. I got up.

"Trust me, Kristena. You are not alone in this. I will prove to you that I am a friend. I'm going to tell you something," he said. "Mr. Narchese has been asking me what we are talking about. Don't worry. I told him this is all confidential. He also thinks you are wasting your math talents by not applying to colleges. I told him he was wrong. And I told him if he ever asks me about you again, I'll report him to the principal."

My hands were folded. I waited to hear more from Dr. Toussaint. For a moment, he didn't feel like a counselor. He looked more like a shadow.

The room suddenly stopped feeling like a psychologist's office. It was now like a closed bedroom or a swing set in a lonely park where two kids talk in secret.

"Are you having breathing problems?" he asked.

My hard, tense face softened. My voice became natural as I spoke.

"I'm breathing ok, but I want to tell you this in case the problems come back and I don't make it," I said. "That kindergarten teacher I told you about... I had the biggest crush on him. I spent months writing a poem for him. But he just laughed."

"He didn't just laugh at you, did he?" Dr. Toussaint asked.

"He told me it was terrible," I cried. "I thought I wrote my best poem and he still thought it was terrible. He said, 'If you keep writing poems, you'll stay a nobody. You won't have any chance at being somebody.' All the other kids called me a baby. It hurt. I don't know why."

"You were very young," he said. "You had deep feelings for someone who insulted you in front of other children. He himself turned away from you. So you let him get to you for years, and you buried it with work."

I nodded.

"Mr. Narchese reminds you of him, doesn't he?" he asked.

"I hate Mr. Narchese. I hate my kindergarten teacher," I said.

"Why do you hate them? No matter how much they try, no one can control your life if you don't let them," he said. "I know Mr. Narchese did this to you and so did your Kindergarten teacher. We want people like them to be punished for hurting us. We want them to know they were wrong. But that's not your responsibility. You owe them nothing. How do you make yourself happy? Don't live as someone you're not. Otherwise, you may as well not have lived at all. It's as if you died, before you really died."

\* \* \*

After the burial ceremony was over, it was just Acia and me at Lam's grave. I wrote one last note on a card and placed it on his grave.

*Dear Lam,*

*In my world, it is 3:15 am. I can't sleep. So I am writing this to say hello.*

*Wherever you are, I hope you're sleeping as well as you did here*

*on earth.*

*Maybe you're not asleep. Maybe you're far more awake than you've ever been.*

*What time is it in your world?*

*We'll meet again. It'll be where there's no more worlds between us.*

*Love,*

*Kristena*

"I miss him so much," Acia said, as we walked home together.

"Poor Lam. I'm sorry for all the things I never gave him."

I told her that is the last thing he would want. I reminded her of the time she told me to never feel sorry for yourself. I told her that if I was Lam and wrote a card, my parting words would be this:

*Dear Mama,*

*You loved me every day. You did more than accept me for who I was. You adored me like a little star. You celebrated my life every day. That is how you treated me in life, and that is how, I know, you want to treat me in death.*

*You were the lady God chose for me as my mama before I was born.*

*You were my best friend.*

*You honored the life that was more important to you than your own life.*

*I don't need you to tell me that you loved me. In the way you valued me, I always knew that.*

*Love,*

*Lam*

I went home and cried harder than I cried for anything in my life. The pain was strongest in the quiet moments. I had to write things down. I kept looking for meaning in all this, and finding none. So I did what I always did. I wrote.

My grades dropped that final semester. The valedictorian was another boy. He gave a great speech but it was long.

If I had given the speech, I would've made it short and simple:

"Time is a gift. Don't miss the chances to live out your dreams.

There is a chance for every good wish you have."

Mom and Dad asked Acia to stay with us in the days after Lam's death.

I missed all the college deadlines, but I did enroll in the local writing school.

Acia spent more time with our family as the years went by. She became a family friend. In turn, Acia would lift me up many times. When I was down, Acia would always remind me of the gift of language that I have. It was something Lam could never have.

"Keep writing, and read out loud. He'll hear you," she would say. "You may not hear him, just like when he was with us, but I believe he will hear you."

So I kept putting all my feelings onto paper. I focused on that. I worked odd jobs here and there to fill in the other times. I always looked forward to moments when I could write.

I don't know if I ever came to the full meaning of why Lam was gone so quickly. It just got more like bits and pieces of a puzzle.

Anyway, that's to be expected. Writing is a journey. It's a process.

It's not a simple solution with one right answer like a math problem.

I met my husband a few years later in a writing workshop. It's pure joy to have a companion read with me and talk about books with me all day long.

Together with Acia, we started a non-profit organization to hold writing workshops and other classes for kids with disabilities. We called it Chance and Little Star. We put them in real jobs, not just in a classroom. We made sure we hired the best teachers and job coaches. Our motto was: "Everyone deserves a chance and a little star to guide them."

Mine was Lam.

I'll be honest. It wasn't all perfect. We struggled with rent and food, and will probably still struggle. But I don't complain. This was the path I chose. These were the consequences I accepted. I had the warmth of my books and my feelings on paper. I treasure each of my adventures in writing. Each day I discover new things about myself that can only come through writing.

Most importantly, I never had another breathing problem again.

But if I'm ever in doubt, I think of those beautiful evenings at that home I visited as a teenager. I cannot forget the heartache that made my decision to choose this path. I would not trade this happiness for anything. That is all I needed in life.

So when my parents call to ask me how I'm doing, I say, "I'm doing great."

Once in a while, they ask if I think about Lam. I still say, "Yes."

What they are really asking me is if I've recovered yet? The answer to that is no. But they will not hear the smallest whimper from me. Because they know what I'll say next.

Recover from Lam? Recover from my most special friendship? Recover from finding my own breath again? Recover from my deepest appreciation of life?

No, and I hope I never will.

# About the Author

Joseph Legaspi's blended writing style reflects his diverse background and interests in both fiction and non-fiction. He wrote for *The Knight News* College Newspaper at Queens College in New York and has worked extensively as a grant writer and as an educator for the City of New York's America Reads Literacy Program.

His love of romantic literature started from reading Dickens and his love of science came from counting stars (cheesy, yes, but true). Somewhere, somehow, the two interests merged and he began writing romantic sci-fi.

# About the Publisher

Story Shares is a nonprofit focused on supporting the millions of teens and adults who struggle with reading by creating a new shelf in the library specifically for them. The ever-growing collection features content that is compelling and culturally relevant for teens and adults, yet still readable at a range of lower reading levels.

Story Shares generates content by engaging deeply with writers, bringing together a community to create this new kind of book. With more intriguing and approachable stories to choose from, the teens and adults who have fallen behind are improving their skills and beginning to discover the joy of reading. For more information, visit storyshares.org.

Easy to Read. Hard to Put Down.

# Notes

www.ingramcontent.com/pod-product-compliance
Lightning Source LLC
Chambersburg PA
CBHW071227170626
46809CB00005BA/1966